WHAT'S INSIDE

Christine Lee-Schaffer

A NOTE TO THE READER

The views and opinions expressed in this book solely those of the author, and are not meant to replace the advice of your health care provider. Any questions or concerns you may have about your physical or mental wellbeing should be addressed with a competent, licensed health care professional.

WHAT'S INSIDE
Christine Lee-Schaffer

ISBN: 978-0-9861558-0-2

Book Design by Taylor Barnes / L7studio.com

Printed in the United States of America

About the Author

Christine Lee-Schaffer received her Doctor of Pharmacy from the University of the Pacific School of Pharmacy in Stockton, California, and was granted a Bachelor of Science in Clinical Laboratory Science from the University of Nevada, Reno. She is licensed by both the California and Nevada State Boards of Pharmacy. She is also a Board Certified Pharmacotherapy Specialist, and a licensed clinical laboratory scientist.

Dr. Lee-Schaffer founded Optimal Life as the natural outgrowth of her association with American Health Care, which she co-founded in 1986. American Health Care specializes in delivering patient-centric pharmacy benefit, population health, and therapy management programs that emphasize clinical excellence. She also developed proprietary software for virtual medical records that is used by hospitals across the country. She is the program director for the company's pharmacy residency program and co-founded the United American Pharmacy Network. Dr. Lee-Schaffer is affiliated with the American College of Managed Care Pharmacy, the American College of Clinical Pharmacy, the American Society of Health System Pharmacists and the Academy of Managed Care Pharmacy.

When not at work, Christine enjoys the company of her family, maintains her black belt in Taekwondo and loves to run. She serves on the board of the Juvenile Diabetes Research Foundation Northern California Inland Chapter, and has served on the boards of several consulting companies, as well as human rights advocacy groups for the mentally disabled.

You may contact the author at info@optimalife.net.

Acknowledgment

There are so many people who have helped support me with love to write this book, but first and foremost are my two children, Jacqueline and Charles. Their unconditional love provides me with the strength to move mountains.

I would also like to thank Sherill Conley Rohde for assistance with everything from ideas, to business, or simply making sure I eat lunch. Her friendship and enthusiasm remind me that we can change lives by giving people knowledge. Thank you so very much.

CONTENTS

Introduction

This book provides individuals the freedom to realize who they are, and remind them of the limitless power that resides deep inside each and every one of us. I want to empower people, to inspire confidence and courage, to let them know that they (we) can make our own decisions and direct our lives, to be what we want it to be. It's time to take back our power and decision-making that has been so directed by society, traditions, a parent, spouse, and even options for health care, and bring forth our desires so that we can manifest a miraculous life.

This book has been in the making for years without my conscious knowledge. It usually takes some type of catalyst or event to draw out the person we are meant to be when we are not being our true self. The signs are there, but until we stop to see what's inside, we only notice small signs and pay little attention to what they may or may not mean.

So, I was living my life, working on health books and running my disease management company, trying to find new ways to help individuals understand what they need to do to take care of themselves and why it is so important to do it. But the questions I found myself asking them started to do a 180 degree turn. I started to ask myself the same questions. I was always so consumed with helping people that I was not looking inside to see what I needed. The scary part of this was I thought I had it all. The beauty is that there is always an equal and opposite side to everything. My desire to help others led me to turning my own life around to a point that I was willing to take an honest look at myself from the inside out.

There is a moment we realize that we are so important to ourselves that we start loving ourselves more by looking inside, seeing what is good for us, and knowing that what is good for us will be good for others. We start to take back our authority and empower ourselves when we concentrate on who we really are, what we really like, what brings us joy, and begin to bring these things into our lives! The more we start listening to ourselves, the true inner core–our essence–we being it, meaning ourselves, an accelerated momentum of "I am in charge" starts to open up new possibilities for our lives that were always there but dormant.

We start to be aligned with our mind, body and soul. Allowing us to listen to our higher self because we are not allowing someone else/society to distract us so much that our thoughts are filled with everyone else's thoughts.

The freedom and power that comes from being you is a gift that everyone desires and has to have. This book will draw out what's inside and define your individualism and that who we are is much more than our physical mind and body. We are spiritual beings that have the power to do anything.

What's inside? Let this book show you.

CHAPTER ONE
Conditioning

Conditioning is a process in which the frequency or predictability of a behavioral response is increased through reinforcement. The question is, "what reinforced our response"? This is what should be examined from the inner person to see are we conditioned to respond a certain way by the things we spend our time on: television, people at the office, family, religious settings, or labels that have been put on us by other people. Do you even know if your thoughts are conditioned and which ones? Have you ever given a response that felt uncomfortable because it was just following everyone else? Well, I think all of us at one time or another have followed others whether it was the right thing to do or not. So as you start your journey through this book with this first chapter, it is to reveal who you really are. All 16 chapters will bring forth the unique person inside of you, and there will be an a-ha moment of certainty – of "I always knew". This book is intended to bring out the best person you are, so be true to yourself as you read, and I promise you will discover many things just as I have while writing it.

Traditions are probably one of the strongest influences in our life because they have been reinforced through many generations without question. Haven't you heard people say, "I do it this way because my mother or father did it this way", not questioning if the behavior is right or wrong? The cycle gets repeated and passed down from generation to generation. But just because our parents did it and believed it doesn't make it true, right or useful. This is not to say that there aren't some traditions that are beneficial. If a certain way of doing something saves time, gives joy and love, or improves things, then that's good! What I am talking about here is the conditioning of the mind that holds us in a negative environment where poverty, illness, unhappiness, jealousy, greed, racism and so on have become the status quo and for the most part go without question.

The time is now. We must be willing to rethink our stories and tell them from a place of inspired learning, where the past becomes a teaching tool. We hear some say that "we must remember where we come from", but I say what if we don't like where we come from? This is not to say that the past is useful to prevent a repeat of wrongdoing, but when we dwell in it, stew in it, harboring unhealed emotions which inspire us to anger, hurt and un-forgiveness then the past is no longer useful. If we continue to tell the same stories the past is destined to be repeated. Therefore, we cannot be inundated with the same negative story because it will become part of our experience and the cycle will continue. What you focus on you will get.

I feel it is important to take a moment to reexamine our beliefs about a thing, a person or a culture. If we have any type of judgments about these things, then it is necessary to take another look and ask ourselves, "Where did these beliefs originate"? I have to say that I have fallen prey to conditioning. All through my youth, my mother told me that I should become a doctor or go into the medical field, and she would always finish the thought with, "you can do anything if you put your mind to it". Well, I was fortunate that I like to help people so I went into the medical field. Then when I had children, what do you think I said? "You can be any kind of doctor you want. There are lots of choices in different specialties and remember, you can do anything if you put your mind to it". I think that last phrase was there because medicine is harder than hard (please excuse me, but shit describes it better, and that is the truth.) So, both my children went to medical school. One wanted to be there. The other did not, but obeyed me because I was the mom and she loved me. It was my conditioning to tell my children this, but following this conditioning ate away at me as I realized that my daughter did not want to be in medical school. Still, after all the years of hard, tortuous work she was not going to give up because I always told her, "you can do anything if you put your mind to it". I realized that if she was doing what she loved, no matter how hard, it would not feel so torturous. The point is that you need to examine how you influence people, especially the ones you love. Is it for their benefit or simply your belief system reflecting what you want the outcome to be? Oh boy! Sometimes the truth just pierces your heart, but the truth is right and we should follow that.

Labeling or branding is another way of conditioning to direct you into a thought or belief that others want you to believe. We see this all the time with commercials, religious typecasting, controlling bosses, and sometimes our spouses who want to steer us in whatever direction fits best for them.

We see whole groups of people responding to words that have been used for decades to describe a particular group. The words are used to degrade, shame and disempower a group or individual. The person responding to the word has been conditioned to believe that the word used refers to him or her in some way, for they feel it necessary to defend, take offense or get upset by the word. The same is true for the individuals using such words. They too believe that the word does in fact describe that particular person or group. I say it is all conditioning. The person using the word has elicited the desired response from the person they've intended to hurt – mission accomplished. The individual that feels offended by the word has also been conditioned to respond in this way. As we watch those before us get upset and feel diminished by the simple use of a word, we follow suit without question and the cycle continues. This addresses both parties, the one using the word and the one reacting to the word. This is then reinforced in the media and by those who believe it to be true.

There isn't one thing we believe that shouldn't come into question, especially if it infringes upon how another group, culture or individual may behave. If we feel it is our duty to police the universe then we have missed the mark. It is people who misinterpret, misunderstand, and are misinformed who speak the loudest, who are the first to judge, and cite the sources that validate their hatred and judgment – all in the name of love they say, but it never feels like love. Then the phrase becomes "tough love". Love isn't tough. If someone says that it is then they are not talking about love.

We see and experience tradition and conditioning in the way we eat. Have you ever seen a commercial that invites you to visit the produce section of a grocery store, with words like, "go directly to the delicious fruit and vegetable section where you will see beautifully colored, mouth-watering fruit that helps you look younger, and leaves your skin and body feeling good through the nutrients and water they supply?" This is a true statement, but it's not what you see in commercials. Oh no, what you see is a beautiful woman with a knockout body eating a double-decker hamburger with the ketchup dripping as she takes another bite of it. Who is really looking at the hamburger? You aren't, and that's the point. It's about attaching sex or good feeling when you eat the hamburger. You're thinking I would like to see her body without clothes. In real life, after a few years of continually eating like that, you really don't want to see her body anymore, and that's the truth as well.

We have become accustomed to bad eating habits because of tradition. We eat too much because it is customary when a big dinner is prepared for you, especially on Sundays or holidays. For example, Aunt Suzy pours you another glass of wine even though you have had enough because it is a holiday tradition. At what point do you start to listen to yourself and decide how much your body really wants? Drinking alcohol is also a conditioned response. Upon taking our first sip of alcohol we may have gagged, choked, or wanted to get sick. Some knew it was not the thing for them and never had the desire to try it again. For others, it would be a just matter of time before they acquired the taste for alcohol by conditioning their taste buds to like it. Simultaneously, commercials showing how much fun it is to drink reinforce the behavior. They show fit, young, attractive friends having a blast together against a picture-perfect backdrop on the beach, in a backyard or other fun-filled setting. The message is that you will be perceived as cool or with the in-crowd if you consume alcohol. Commercials never show you the long term effects of excessive drinking and what it does to our bodies.

The same scenario applies to cigarette smoking. You will see the same backdrop with fit, young, attractive people selling the idea of being cool, hip or sexy. But they never mention the long terms effects, or the stench in your clothes, hair, house, or in a room and, more importantly, your breath (my opinion). We have been conditioned to tolerate, accept and embrace beliefs that threaten and jeopardize our health and the health of those around us.

I say it is time to do away with our outdated beliefs that hold us back from dreaming and living the best life we can imagine. It doesn't matter what our parents and their parents did or didn't do. If the life that we are living is not what we desire and isn't benefiting us and those around us, then what good are those beliefs if they are not life affirming?

French researcher, Alphonso Bertillon, said, "One can only see what one observes, and one can observe only things that are already in the mind." In other words, if the mind has been conditioned to confrontation, struggle, prejudices, and sadness then the individual can only see these things in his/her world. This will be the topic of conversation. The programs they seek out on the TV or internet will reflect this, and so their life experiences are reinforced by conditioning, and is reinforced by media in what they choose to watch for they have created it by default.

Anything to which we give real meaning or power in our lives is created by us, by our belief system. And so we must protect and evaluate our belief system to see how much of it is conditioned and where did the conditioning come from.

People in the United States spend an average of 5 hours and 11 minutes each day watching television. The average child watches 1,480 minutes or 24.6 hours of television each week. The average American youth spends 900 hours per year in school, but watches about 1,200 hours of television yearly, and will see 16,000 30-second commercials. By the age of 18, children will see 150,000 violent acts on TV. With these statistics it is obvious where the conditioning comes from. Now what are we willing to do about what influences us?

Human conditioning: We have the power to change every aspect of our lives for we have been conditioned to believe certain things. We can also recondition ourselves to believe something that will be more beneficial for our lives and those around us.

Affirmation

The Human Condition

- I am the master of my circumstances.
- I am in the flow of goodness.
- I am in the flow of the best that I can imagine.
- I see the beauty in every moment.
- I am willing to begin again.
- I am willing to think a new better feeling.
- I am willing to listen to my heart's desires.
- I am aligned with all the blessings that are available.
- I am aligned with the power of prayer.
- My condition is improving in every moment.

CHAPTER TWO
Food for Life

Eating provides us with the nutrients to sustain a healthy body. But it should also energize every fiber of our being, help us function at our absolute best, and inspire us to new levels of awareness. Most people live to eat instead of eating to live. The majority of food choices that are made come down to condition and tradition from our parents, their parents, and generations before, just like the cultural traditions that are centered around special foods on special occasions that are cause for a feast. It is a tradition, therefore no one questions it, as it has been the theme for years, even decades. Families sit down to enjoy good conversation and a great meal. In the midst of it all, no one considers what they are actually eating. They watch their midsection expand and their health start to decline all in the name of a good meal, just like the generations before. They do not ask one question as to the validity of the nutritional content of the food, most of which is high in fat and carbohydrates, but boy does it taste good. We have been conditioned to love these cultural foods. Through years of programming, our taste buds have learned to love them and actually crave them.

It is time we think of food for life, to provide health and nutrition to our body, mind and soul. The majority of the food we have come to love by condition and tradition are far from keeping us healthy. Eating a healthy diet is one of the best and most direct ways we can influence our health, such as cholesterol levels, blood pressure, asthma, weight, colon cancer, heart disease and so on. So if we know this, why is it so difficult to choose foods that we know will provide our body with the perfect life-giving energy necessary for a more healthy body, that will fill us with life force, and restore our bodies to perfect balance, allowing for natural health and healing? After all the body knows best. Our body knows what to do to get us in balance, but we must do our part by giving it the proper nutrients to do so as opposed to food that when eaten for extended periods of time has the potential to cause sickness, disease and weight issues.

When we deal with our emotional problems by eating to mask the discomfort, we are operating on automatic by doing what we know. In the past, a child would get candy as a reward for being good at the doctor's office, and if we were lucky our parents would take us out for ice cream. Now we've come to expect some form of treat based on our behavior, by being a good little boy or girl. We have an emotional attachment to an outside conditioned response that we feel makes us feel better at that moment we consume the food. How often do we find ourselves reaching for the ice cream or a chosen dessert at the moment of feeling some form of discomfort – be it a bad day or hurt and upset feelings? It is all learned behavior. Instant gratification like this is the catalyst for an unhealthy body because it produces long-term effects that are not addressed. How long do you think your body will tolerate it?

"Your youth is your grace period."

We must come to a place where we are capable of asking ourselves, "Why am I continuing to sabotage my health and wellbeing?" Each person may have a different answer, but it all boils down to the same thing – condition and tradition. After a while we become more and more complacent, and our eating habits go global; the majority has embraced processed foods as the norm. All foods that are white are processed, and are essentially a drug because they come with side effects, and are just as addictive as any illegal drug – not to mention that they have been manufactured, and purposely created to cause addiction. We must ask ourselves are we eating the way the majority of people do based on condition and tradition, or are we making healthy choices because we wish to live a more healthy lifestyle in mind, body and soul, so that we can enjoy life to the fullest?

You have a choice. It is not necessary to do what everyone else does, leading to a life and body riddled with physical ailments that could have been avoided just by making healthier choices. We know that processed foods are devoid of nutritional value, not to mention they cause an increase in chronic diseases. We are either part of the system or we are observing it from afar and making better choices, as we listen to the all-knowing authentic self from within that guides us to a healthy body.

Many of us look outside ourselves for someone to give us accurate information, but we can no longer trust others to determine what's best for us. I was always taught that if you don't make decisions for yourself, other people will make them for you, and it is usually not in your best interest. Should you trust yourself or trust strangers who are probably benefiting from your wrong decisions and lack of education in a given area?

Would you water a dying plant with soda, sugary juices or artificial sweeteners that are filled with chemicals instead of life-giving water? Would you continue eating and drinking the same foods that may have led to your illness? How could anything change in your body when you're not changing what you put in it? When you align your body with good nutritional food, the goodness provides you with energy and clarity that lead to the next step in your recovery. A healthy diet should be just what the doctor ordered – nowadays it's medication, which are more chemicals in the body.

With this all said, let's talk a little about the influence society has put on the family and you, as an individual. At every turn we are bombarded with propaganda. The sole purpose of these companies' commercials is to misinform and mislead us as to the true nature and purpose of the products being advertised. We are told that these products are good for us, that they are beneficial to our health. As a child we don't have much to say about what we will or will not eat, especially if our parents were more interested in taste over quality. In most families it was tradition and condition. If our parents and grandparents ate a particular food or foods then more often than not we would eat the same food. In some cases it comes down to what a family could afford. There are families that eat dessert after every meal and those that have a soda or a sweet beverage with every meal. I say it is learned behavior – monkey see, monkey do. We learn to cook by watching our parents. So, some of the ailments that we may have witnessed our parents and grandparents experience may be directly linked to their eating habits, which is tied into their belief system thus the thing we call hereditary.

It has been drilled into our belief system that milk is good for us, but it's debatable that milk from cows, goats, etc., really is good for us. Is it a moral

dilemma or a nutritional one? I believe the decision should be based on the nutritional benefits that milk may or may not have. But for generations now, we've been told that milk is good for us. Now we have been conditioned to believe milk is a necessary part of our daily diet...mission accomplished! We have bought into this concept as truth, and now the milk producers have conditioned several generations of families into believing that they need milk. This is the case for the majority of the foods consumed in American households. If we take a close look at typical American food products we find they have no nutritional value or health benefits at all.

When we are preoccupied with the outside world, and trying to juggle all of our responsibilities - parents and single mothers and fathers trying to make a living – it is hard to find the time to investigate what is being put into our foods. Most of us trust that food manufacturers have our highest good in mind when describing the nutritional value of their product. But often we are too busy or too lazy to discover if it's true, so we just take their word for it and continue living and eating "stuff", believing we are doing right by our families and loved ones based on someone else's word. It then becomes the least important thing because we have tradition for that; we believe the food manufacturers, so we don't have to think about it...just go with the flow. That is until we contract some illness that would have us reexamine our lives. The word "contract" refers to an agreement between two parties. Consider this when we are not taking responsibility for our health. We enter into a non-verbal contract with the companies that are producing "stuff" for us to eat. I can't call it food because the word food refers to a nutritious substance that people or animals eat. Because we now have this non-verbal contract, we are agreeing to eat whatever they put into the perfect package without question. It is when we do not question what we are eating that we are destined to enter a contract with an illness that will sneak up on us sometimes without warning. Now we are in a contract with the illness. We have entered a non-verbal agreement with the illness to be sick because we were not interested in what we were putting into our bodies.

Now this "stuff" we call food is being marketed in a way that wants us to take the advertisers' word for it. They get an actor or some well-known person to push their product, and because we admire this individual we want to emulate them. So, if they are drinking milk then it must be OK because so-and-so is drinking it–meaning that it must be good for us.

Food manufacturers spend millions of dollars to employ scientists to invent ways to make their products taste better. Psychological studies are also done on the texture, color and smell to see what combination is the most appealing to people. Very little effort is made to make food healthier. The sugar, caffeine, and other ingredients that I am unaware of will send you on a rollercoaster of sugar and caffeine highs. When you finally come down and grab another cookie or candy bar, the manufacturers say "cha-ching", and your body says diabetes, heart attack or excess weight, and your soul's vibrations slow down. The mind, body and soul are all connected. You can't separate them no matter how hard you try. With this in mind, how important to you are the traditional foods that you know are not good for you? Are you going the break the mold of diabetes in your family? Are you going to break the bonds of obesity in your family? Are you going to start anew and teach your loved ones how to do better? Or are you going to take the easy route and have outsiders and society dictate what is best for you? Look inside your neighborhood grocery store and you will see what society thinks is good for your health.

So what is it going to be? If you are going to align yourself with health, there must be a shift in consciousness. Do not let the outside world dictate your decisions about food. We must be inspired to eat healthier foods, with good nutritional value. Healthy food choices will give you maximum energy needed for body, mind and soul. If you believe that your body is a temple for the soul, spirit or energy (whatever you wish to call it), then it must be important to keep it healthy.

AFFIRMATION TWO

Food for Life: The purpose of food for life is that we might have the best quality of life possible, supporting longevity and good health, not to mention we will feel and look better.

Affirmation

Food for Life

- I am choosing food that uplifts me.
- I am choosing nutritionally sound food.
- I am choosing food that gives me energy.
- I am choosing to eat for good health.
- I am choosing to feel better by eating better.
- I am choosing to have an ideal weight by making better choices.
- I am choosing my food as a medicine.
- I am choosing food that empowers me in my mind, body and soul.
- I am choosing food that inspires me to emotional balance.
- I am choosing to incorporate fresh fruits and vegetables on a daily basis.

CHAPTER THREE

What do you Believe?

What do you believe? Why do you believe it? Where did this belief come? It is very important to discover why we have or do not have the life we wish to experience. First we must get to a place where we are seeking something more. If we are unhappy with some part of our lives then we must be willing to investigate our belief system. If we just continue to complain about the things that we are unhappy about we remain tied to those same things (life experiences). These are the questions that we must ask ourselves in order to evaluate our belief system. The very fact that we are here on the planet and have parents, partners, friends and family means that we have picked up a few beliefs that may no longer serve us. We may also hold beliefs we are not conscious of. Every decision we make consciously or unconsciously stems from our beliefs about it. Our belief system also directs our perception of the truth, and this truth whether right or wrong acts as our framework for life the same way a blueprint is the framework of a house. Once the house is framed the only way to change the floorplan is to tear it down and rebuild, but this requires action. This means we must ask the Three Big Questions to see if the motives behind what we believe are based in truth: what do I believe? Why do I believe it? Where did this belief come from? The answers must align us with the life we want to live, and the person we wish to be.

Our beliefs are determined by our behavior, the words we use, and the thoughts we think. It is bigger than genes alone, or brain chemicals and hormones. The brain is a sponge that accepts input without filters, whether good or bad, and sorts that input according to our belief system. This influences how you will react or not react, accept as truth or not truthful.

Why is it that sometimes we do things that we shouldn't do when we know better? Is it that we are rebellious, think differently and can't help ourselves, or just do not know what to do? Somehow a message was programmed into our brain that decreases the seriousness or level of interest to take action. This creates a complacent belief pattern.

I believe we want to do the right things in life. So why is it so difficult for us to take control of our lives, perform well at work, lose weight, exercise, and take care of ourselves or our loved ones? These lifestyle choices are all under our control, but if we believe that consequences do not always apply to every situation or are not so bad that they can't wait, we will not always act in our best interest, or a loved one's best interest. Society has programmed us into complacency which causes us to do nothing. After all if we don't want to cook there is always unhealthy fast food. If we need money we get an advance on our paychecks. There is no need to be responsible. Why excel at work if you will get a paycheck anyway? There's no need to walk to work if you have a car. You get the idea. All these comforts and choices are masterminded by people who are becoming wealthy off your choices. Once we fall into complacency our minds are primed to be non-directional. This sets up an environment that allows manipulation of the masses to be swayed in any direction for another's comfort, convenience, power, greed or wealth. Complacency has been society's biggest downfall and is our biggest downfall. When we become complacent, the desire to direct our lives is lost, and the power to do so may feel non-existent. Instead, we sit there waiting to be told what to do or what to like. Remember the commercial, "Winston tastes good like a cigarette should"? How many people smoked Winston because they were told it tasted good? And how many started smoking Winston because it was said to be a good tasting cigarette? This conditioning is the power of listening to others instead of listening to the power within. Do not be fooled into thinking that complacency exists in only one area of your life and does not affect other areas. How many areas do you think smoking Winston cigarettes affected: health, money, the effects of secondhand smoke on your loved ones, smelly clothes and so on. Complacency is a mindset that robs you of your power and individualism. The decisions we make allow us to change our thought patterns if we desire this. Going forward you will see that when we question why we make the decisions we do, we regain our ability to take control of our thoughts, allowing us to make better decisions and become empowered to have any and everything we want.

We feel justified by our beliefs. Justified is defined as: to demonstrate or prove to be just, right or valid. I believe this means we are living a life, wanted or unwanted, based on what we believe because we believe it. Our belief makes it real for us and the proof is in the pudding: our life experience justifies the belief. What we believe becomes real for us in our mind, body and soul. How do we get our thoughts and power back so that they manifest what we believe? All of this ties into the understanding of who we truly are. This is how powerful we are. We have the power to call something into existence that did not exist before.

"Call those things that be not as though they were."

To believe you can create something begins with a thought. If you believe that what you think is possible, you start to set the motion of that thought into existence. For example, Bill Gates and Paul Allen formed a partnership called Microsoft. They had a thought that evolved into a huge vision – a computer on every desk and in every home. People may have thought they were nuts, but history speaks for itself. What about the thought that you want to build a home someday, or a company, or go to college when no one in your family has ever gone, or run a marathon after breaking your neck? Again, if you believe it is possible, you will align yourself in a manner that will make it happen.

What do you believe? Do you believe that you are healed? Are you acting like the thing you wish to manifest? (be different; name it want you want it to be, not what it is). What do you believe? Do your eating habits align with what you believe? If you want to lose weight but you are eating food that contradicts your desire, there is no alignment, no agreement. If you are talking about believing in getting better, then your thoughts must be in alignment with getting better. Eat foods that set you up for the belief you have about losing weight, then translate it to every area of your being. It cannot be isolated, and as the path is repeated it begins to form a healthier habit.

Do you believe you are going to have a health condition because of heredity? However you respond to this will be the truth. You have it because you believe it. I will tell you this: everybody has what they believe. As a young child my mother believed that I must be allergic to penicillin because she was. In fact, she seemed to be allergic to everything, and the more she said, "I am allergic to everything", the more she would have a reaction to everything. Her words became her reality. I never believed that I was allergic to anything and guess what, I am not and this applies to penicillin.

Belief is doing. Right now, you are doing what you believe. Everyone in poverty is doing what they believe. Those that are choosing chemotherapy are doing what they believe. Those choosing alternative medicine are doing what they believe. Belief is key.

What do you believe you are worth? Minimum wage, college education, owning a company, being a millionaire or billionaire. What do you believe you are worth? Do you believe you are worthy of a healthy life, so you can live without illness? Do you believe that? Do you believe it is possible? Look around you. There are people doing it. So, yes, it is possible. Choose to be the example for others. That is the purpose of all of us is to be an example for others. So what is your purpose? Is your belief about your life strong enough to be an example, not only for your own health and well-being, but to give strength to others? Whatever a person believes becomes possible. The house you have is because you believe you can have it. It is the only reason you have it.

What do you believe? Do you believe you are going to get better? Do you believe in miracles? Do you believe the body knows what to do and how to heal itself? Do you believe that you are capable of finding a remedy? Do you believe that you can wake up on a regular basis feeling good? Do you believe you can feel this way all the time? Our future is designed and shaped by our belief system and this will determine if our positive thoughts, dreams, or miracles will come to fruition. Yesterday's thoughts are today's reality. Our inspired thoughts are the path to freedom that will knock down any belief system that is holding us back, if we allow it. All thoughts are creative and if we allow ourselves to focus on inspirational, happy and uplifting thoughts our lives will begin to change. We must hold onto these thoughts long enough to gain some momentum because it will trump any contradictory thought /belief system that says that we can't. It is our choice, to be inspired and break through to manifest our thoughts, or let the belief system around us dictate and confine us to a life that is less fulfilling. So, what do you believe?

What do you believe? What we believe will determine what we think, feel and experience. If we are not satisfied with our lives, all we need do is change our belief about it.

Affirmation

What do you Believe?
- I believe in magic.
- I believe in miracles.
- I believe in love.
- I believe that I am the healer.
- I believe that I am connected to the healing powers of the universe.
- I believe in the unlimited potential of goodness and greatness.
- I believe in peace.
- I believe that I am all that I am meant to be in this moment.
- I believe in the healing power of love.
- I believe in the divine consciousness where all is well and perfect.
- I believe in perfect timing.
- I believe in the healing power of my body for it is perfect just the way it is.

CHAPTER FOUR

Who are we?

We are more than blood, flesh and bones. We hear in religious teaching that we are spiritual beings having a physical experience. I say if this is the case then let's prove it. I believe the first step to uncovering this truth is to contemplate the true nature of our being. We know that the body is capable of healing itself from all sorts of ailments, no matter what the condition may be. We have heard of healings of all kinds – we call them miracles. I say it is an individual deciding to become one with the vision of perfect health, the healed self in mind, body and soul (the body must follow the mind). One spiritual teaching advises us to "know thyself". How does the body know what to do? How does the body heal a wound? If we are to believe that we are just flesh, blood and bones, then how is it possible that a woman experiences superhuman strength? We hear accounts of the seemingly impossible, and yet there is the proof that a woman was capable of lifting a car to save her child or a loved one. I say in that moment she was completely aligned with the desire to do so. There were no doubts or contradictory thoughts to the contrary. In a different setting this act might have been impossible, but under the right circumstances all is possible when aligned with the truth of our nature.

We do not need to go to such lengths to prove that we are more than what we once thought (only human). Let's take our thoughts. If we are willing to look at our lives, we will soon see the part that our thoughts are playing in shaping our experiences. I would encourage you to reread the chapter on beliefs. Once we are willing to assume responsibility for our thoughts, we will begin to see the potential power we possess. We are powerful when we have a thought about our lives in mind, body and soul, hold our attention on that thing, and before long it becomes our experience.

We come to the realization that we see what we expect to see: our home, relationships (or lack thereof), the type of car we drive, etc. Haven't you thought of someone and within moments they called you, or you encounter them soon after the thought? I am sure that everyone can relate to making a right turn instead of a left while driving because you instinctively knew it was the right way to go. How about turning into a parking lot and knowing that there will be a parking space exactly where you would like it? All of this is expectation and alignment of our thoughts with our desires. Some may chalk it up to coincidence, but to say so disempowers us. It is no coincidence. People who do not believe in perfect timing will also find it difficult to believe that a person can possess extraordinary internal power. Because of this they may believe coincidence explains an event for which there is no explanation. I believe that there is no such thing as coincidence. If we believe that we are so much more than flesh, blood and bones, the mere fact that a woman can lift a car off a child cannot be explained. Nor can we explain a person's body being taken over by large, cancerous tumors, given less than 24 hours to live, and then survive. Not only does this individual survive, but she is cured of cancer. In the case of the woman's extraordinary strength, adrenaline alone is not enough to allow her to lift the car off her child. Adrenaline only increases strength as far as a person's existing muscle mass allows. Therefore, these events are miracles, as there is no logical explanation for how they could have occurred.

We may call it being in the perfect zone when our thoughts are so aligned with our desires that they come to fruition. Miracles and miraculous healings happen when we are aligned with the desire to be healed in mind, body and soul. We are much bigger than our behavior. According to some religious teachings the kingdom of heaven is within. I interpret this to mean that God is inside of us, not external to us. What we believe is what will exist, and it exists because it's what we believe. This includes illness, success, and good relationships. It doesn't matter what we believe because our thoughts make it real. It is up to us what we choose to think.

A small child is not tainted with what is man-made until that child is taught. A child believes that anything is possible; many people call this imagination. What we imagine is real because our thoughts dictate what our experiences will be. Everything is lovely to a child until taught otherwise. The possibilities are endless – beautiful, clear, without fear, and existing at that moment of pure loving thoughts. Therefore, we all need to guard our thoughts so that we fill our minds with what is lovely, what we want to be, what our hopes and dreams are, because it sets the path for manifestation. We are the directors of our path and who we want to be. The nature within us will allow things to flourish regardless of whether or not we are being true to ourselves, meaning it is creative in all directions no matter what we are focused on. Our internal life force is directed toward us, expressing our true nature and expanding our horizon to be all that we can be. There is no contradiction in our path and no coincidence when we allow the eternal power to be expressed because it provides the confidence to move forward steadfastly and unwavering regardless of what anyone else's opinion of us may be. All of us are unique with a purpose to why we are here, and this uniqueness is exhilarating and powerful. Once we believe in the power we possess and all its possibilities, the fullness of life that is experienced is endless. I can't express enough the feeling of freedom I have learned when I started allowing the true nature of who I am to manifest. There are no words to describe it.

We are much more, and we may act "less than" for as long as we like, but the ability to be great is always available in each moment with every passing thought. So, who do you wish to be now that you know we are much more than blood, flesh and bone?

Who are you? Who do you want to be? Do you want to be a person of integrity, compassion, perfect health? It is your choice. Decide who you want to be and walk in that direction.

Affirmation

Who Are You?

- I am a spiritual being with access to the universe.
- I am the question and the answer.
- I am a person who shares light and love.
- I am looking for the best life has to offer.
- I am my thoughts and my thoughts are love.
- I am the universe.
- I am the gift.
- I am that I am.
- I am a manifestation of light and love.
- I am pure love; I am humility; I am grace.

CHAPTER FIVE

Mind, Body and Soul

The phrase mind, body and soul is used so frequently today. I am not sure if those that choose to use this phrase have a full understanding of its meaning. I believe this phrase is intended to describe the fullness of being an integrated individual in mind, body and soul. There may be some level of understanding of what is meant by these words, but we will never be fully empowered until we have a full grasp of what it means to be whole.

When we hear the phrase mind, body and soul, or holy trinity - God, the Father and Son – we also hear the meaning that I now believe has been misinterpreted. Some religious teachings say that when two, three or more are gathered then God is present. The teachings say we need at least two others to agree with us in order for God to be present. This may be a problem. What if no one believes what you believe? This implies that it is necessary for another person to agree with you. In my understanding of this phrase it is not necessary for anyone to be in agreement to experience the presence of God – please replace "God" with the word or name that resonates most with you.

We are starting to awaken to this truth that the power of God or the connection to God does not come from a person or a spiritual leader. Some believe that it is a state of consciousness but consciousness is a function of the brain. The brain is an organ and is not the spiritual power. Only the spirit has the ability to inspire and bring powerful knowledge to your brain for understanding, not the other way around. We must come to a place of remembering or to rediscover that it is not a person outside of ourselves. Those outside of you – your sister, brother, husband, wife, priest, rabbi, mother, father or best friend – do not need to be in agreement with you for you to experience the presence and power God. If you believe that access to God or God's power is from a spiritual leader or a person then you are limiting yourself to their human limitations. It is wonderful to admire people for their contribution to society, but who wants to limit God? Why would God put this limitation on us to find a person who could be in complete agreement with mind, body and soul when we are all made to be unique? Our uniqueness is part of God, our spirit. The only way a real connection is made is from within, because no two people can be in complete agreement because they have preoccupations in their own world. What is offered can only be halfhearted. Therefore, the experience of God is very personal, and is experienced in countless ways. So next time you have an a-ha moment, recognize that the spirit was awakening your brain to the inspired answer or power that you needed, not an outside source.

The mind, body and soul concept means there are three states available: mind, body, and soul/spirit. For example, let's say you decide to start a new exercise routine that includes a morning walk. You have decided to start first thing tomorrow morning. This is something you've contemplated for weeks, and now it's time to do it. Your thoughts may go something like this: "Wow, morning has come quickly. I need more sleep." You go over your to-do list in your mind and then you remember the walk you promised yourself you would start today. You must make a choice: do you go for a walk this morning, as promised, or do you sleep longer because today is your last day off before going back to work? You are now having a full discussion with yourself about taking the morning walk. Now two are present for this discussion, and one will win. Will it be the mind and the desire to walk, or the body, feeling tired and needing more sleep? When two or more are gathered within we can also say they become aligned with the desire to walk. When the body obeys the mind they are in alignment.

The illustration above is an example of agreement, but where is the power in this agreement? The body and mind may agree, but for someone to manifest a desire, a healing, or create protection from danger this agreement falls short, because you must be aligned in mind, body and soul. It is when you access the spirit within that you access unlimited power, a power that is so strong that any agreement between your mind and body cannot be broken, a power that can instantaneously change any circumstance, and manifest your desires. When aligned, it can protect you from danger at the blink of an eye. This power comes from our soul/spirit. It is an integral part of our makeup. If you want to access this power, you must realize that you are a spiritual being. Everyone is a spiritual being, and your body houses this spirit.

It is no different than getting in a car. You do not become the car, but you are capable of operating the car because you are familiar with the manual. The manual describes what you can or cannot do with the car. Similarly, when you are here in your body, you are operating the body and, again, someone has taught you the limiting beliefs and purpose of your body. We are taught how to use the body, and usually we are misinformed. Certainly, this is because our parents were misinformed. So, imagine getting into a car and not knowing how to operate it because you do not have the manual. Then someone says that it only goes ten miles per hour because that's what they were told. They never questioned it or tried to go faster. No one has driven 15 or 20 miles per hour because no one has stepped outside the box. No one has questioned what they've been told.

We are much more. The body is lovely, but we understand that the body is just a vehicle like our car. So the body is the vehicle even in religious teaching. You say, "Use me, God. Use me as your vehicle. Let me be your vessel." And so, do not be distracted by the body. I wish for you to empower yourself by first remembering that you are much more than your physical body. You are occupying the car, but you are not the car. You are occupying the body, but you are not the body. I'm sure some of you believe that the body is who you are, and that is why you become weak and helpless because you believe that it is all that you are. That concept in and of itself renders you powerless.

People often try to manifest their dreams using their minds to set goals for success, weight loss, buying a house, and so forth. You might create a list of well thought-out goals, but why do many desires not come to fruition? Unless the mind has some ability to protect its thoughts from the outside influences, the desire peters out. There must be a force which provides a shift in consciousness, of knowing with certainty that the dream can be accomplished.

When you believe you are a spiritual being and you connect to the spirit within, there is a change in you. The essence of your being becomes more confident and more assured. The ability to follow through and make things happen becomes effortless. Accessing the spirit influences or changes the thought patterns in your brain to have certainty. Certainty allows confidence to flow through your brain, which sets the brain up for success. It allows you to think clearly. Anytime you have clarity of thought you know the spirit and mind are aligned. Once you have experienced this, and understand that it came from within, you will want to continue this alignment as much as possible. There is no fear when you are certain, only momentum toward the goal.

The power of our spirit is right here within all of us. Everyone has access at any time. It provides perfect alignment with the body and mind if you would like it. So, where do you want your power to come from?

Mind, Body and Soul: Are you walking the walk, doing what you say you desire in mind, body and soul, and acting like the person you say you want to be?

Affirmation

Mind Body and Soul

- My mind, body and soul are aligned.

- I am aligned with the power.

- I am filled with love in my mind, body and soul.

- I have complete balance with my mind, body and soul.

- I am one with joy in my mind, body and soul.

- I am one with health in my mind, body and soul.

- I am one with abundance (wealth) in my mind, body and soul.

- I am in pure bliss with my mind, body and soul.

- I am one with the creator in my mind, body and soul.

- I am aligned with the truth in my mind, body and soul.

CHAPTER SIX

Whose Responsibility is it?

We are wise enough to know better. We can decide to do something different to make better choices for ourselves. We do not have to pretend that we are powerless before our circumstances. When we are old enough to know better, we do better. As children we may have rules we must follow, but even then we may feel a level of knowing that contradicts that which is being forced upon us. Whatever disempowering habits we've learned as children should no longer matter. We must be willing to take responsibility for our lives. Every aspect of it. What is working or not working is our responsibility. It is interesting that we find different levels of responsibility in different areas of our life. Some may be very responsible about paying bills, but irresponsible in their eating habits, leading to obesity or vice versa. Whatever area is being neglected is due to conditioning from our environment.

It is up to us to flush out what belief created our inability to take action when action is needed. To do so requires us to think independently and objectively. The greater the influence of the person that caused you to accept a certain condition or the strength of their authority, such as a parent, the stronger the barrier to independent thinking. But when you know why you think a certain way, you begin to activate your independent thinking because now you have differentiated yourself from what influenced you. Taking this first step will help you to identify your reasoning or thought patterns that bring about your actions or inaction. This is extremely important because we innately know when we are not doing the right thing which creates discord in our psyche and causes us to be out of alignment.

We can break this down in categories for our lives. Let's start with health. If we are starting out with a healthy body, and then begin listening to conversations about illnesses or hereditary conditions, such as type 2 diabetes, then we start to expect what we now believe is hereditary. I will tell you what is hereditary: the thoughts of our family become hereditary, and therefore our experiences must follow. More often than not if we have the same thought process as our family, then nine times out of ten we will have a similar life experience as our family/parents. If we are looking at our family or our family history of illness, it is our responsibility to educate ourselves. It is our responsibility to ask questions and find out how this originated, and then make a decision as to if we wish to believe it to be our experience or destination. For instance, type 2 diabetes is a condition triggered or made worse by poor food choices and being overweight. As an adult, you choose your food and lifestyle. You have the choice to break the bondage of belief that you will get diabetes because your parents and their parents had diabetes.

I believe in miracles and that anything is possible if we are willing to take responsibility for how we feel about the illness. There may be exceptions to this rule, and even then we still have the power to choose how we wish to think.

It is necessary that we focus on what we give our attention to, particularly regarding our mother, father or siblings. So it is about paying attention to all of that. This is when we start to take responsibility for our lives, for our thoughts, for our experience, so there is a difference. The difference is we get to decide who we want to be, and how we want to be in the world, as opposed to going with the flow, following tradition. As we look at different cultures, we see women who are still treated as second class citizens based on traditions. Some of them wake up and start to think independently rather than accept their situation. They say it is not right that women are treated this way; it does not feel right. The responsibility lies with the individual when they decide that a level of discomfort is no longer tolerable or acceptable. At this point tradition does not make sense.

Then you have those that say, "I am doing it because my parents did it". You have parents that do not say, "I love you" to their child. Then the child grows up and has children of their own, and they do not say "I love you" to their children. If they examine this, they might say, "My mother did not say it to me, so this is how I do it." We might ask them, "How did it make you feel when your parents didn't say it to you?" The response will be that they didn't like it, and yet here they are repeating the pattern, not taking responsibility for breaking a pattern that didn't make them feel good, special or loved.

You are in control of whatever the pattern may be of not taking care of things or allowing an unhealthy condition to continue, whether it is to your family, yourself, a job, or health, you are responsible for it. You know what it is. The question to ask yourself is are you going to allow something in your life that is not right dictate your future, or are you going direct your future, and be responsible? You do have a choice. What's it going to be?

AFFIRMATION SIX

*Whose responsibility is it? We must start
to remember and realize that we have the
power to manifest the best life has to offer.
The first step is taking responsibility for
our thoughts, words and deeds.*

Affirmation

Who's Responsible?

- I am responsible for my health.
- I am responsible for my wealth.
- I am responsible for my wellbeing.
- I am responsible for my thoughts.
- I am responsible for my body.
- I am responsible for my emotional self.
- I am responsible for my behavior and how I interact with the world.
- I am responsible for all the beauty I experience.
- I am responsible for allowing love to flow though me.
- I am responsible for my happiness.
- I am responsible for what I choose to see in the world.
- I am responsible for what I look at.
- I am responsible for my perception.
- I am responsible for myself.

CHAPTER SEVEN

What is There to Fear?

Franklin D. Roosevelt said it best: "The only thing we have to fear is fear itself." Put another way, there is nothing to fear but that to which we give our attention. I believe in some instances fear comes down to a lack of understanding and confidence. It is usually the unhealed residual emotions waiting to be healed/released from our emotional selves. Let's say you're in a new relationship. Your first date went very well and you believe that you are sure to have another one, but there is no follow-up phone call. In that moment you may think that the other person is busy and doesn't have time to call. This is day one. You have told yourself all sorts of reasons why you haven't received a call, and accepted the fact that maybe he or she doesn't want to appear too eager. To add fuel to your fears you may seek the opinion of a friend and they add their well-intended fears to the pot. In this scenario we do not have enough information, and yet we immediately start to question what we could have said or done. I could go on but I feel you get the point.

When we are confident we know that there was nothing that we have done and the reason he or she hasn't called will or will not be revealed at a later date. We are not wandering around like a lost puppy until we get the answer that we believe will bring us closure. I believe as we start to understand our true nature as the manifesters of our own experiences, we will know that the thing we fear is of our own doing, that we have given life to the thing we fear. This means we can remove our attention/focus from the thing we fear, and focus on the goodness, the miracles, the magic and love that life has to offer. We may choose love over anything else. It comes down to the type of questions we are asking. Would it not be better to stabilize ourselves with questions about what is lovely and joyful in our life? What makes us laugh, or what has given us feelings of hope, optimism, peace and excitement in the past? Once we feel better it is easier to ask questions such as, "is it my lack of understanding or lack of education that is making me feel this way?" Is there a different perspective that provides me with better feeling-thoughts, with the sense of feeling unstoppable? When we change our emotions we will find the information we need to turn what gave us the fear sensation into fearlessness. It is not fear or the bogeyman. It is the not knowing or understanding.

Do you remember when you were a child and you had a bad dream or were afraid of something, and your mother or father picked you up, held you, gave you love, told you a story to take your mind off of what gave you the emotion of fear? What happened? It disappeared. Did anything change at that moment? Nothing except your focus. How did that make you feel? Safe? If you want to feel wonderful, change your focus. It does not matter what is causing the fear: a job loss, disappointments, a failed marriage or sickness. Focusing on what is giving you this feeling of fear will freeze your ability to change or overcome it, so change your focus.

Not understanding and not knowing facts or outcomes appears as fear, but it is not. There are times we have fear because we are not doing what we should be doing because we do not know what to do. It is out of not knowing that there is an alternative cancer treatment, alternative solutions to financial problems, or a solution for all issues. It is based on what you have given your attention to. If you believe that chemo is the only answer for cancer because you have not looked outside the box and have not stepped outside the box, then you believe this is all there is. So, it is out of ignorance that appears to be fear. But it is not.

When you have feelings of fear, tune your mind into thinking pleasant thoughts, find something to appreciate, something or someone to change your emotional state. It is very difficult to find a solution when you have internalized negative feelings. Have you ever thought about a person and somehow that person received that thought and gave you a call? Your thoughts made it happen. With this in mind, if you don't change your emotion from fear to love, isn't it possible that you will attract more of what caused the fear because that is what you are focusing on? We must think good and lovely thoughts to get our mind out of the rut of fear. Lovely thoughts allow solutions to the issue to appear because our mind is not cluttered with unwanted and unnecessary fearful thoughts.

There is not one person who has not experienced fear and somehow they overcame what gave them the fear regardless of the outcomes. Knowing this – is fear really real? Can you touch it, smell it, have a conversation with it? Or is it a barometer of our negative feelings out of control? If it is a barometer then we should only use it as such to give us notice that we must shift our focus. Since thoughts can produce things, what gave us the fear needs to be eliminated, or our focus changed at that very moment. Most things you fear will never happen. There are fundamental positive thoughts you can use to turn around the thought of fear and eliminate it. Fundamentals give us certainty to help change our focus because we know those fundamentals are true and give us a reference of stability. As we start to explore this, everyone has basic human fundamentals that we can agree on. Agreeing to questions that you ask yourself helps put your mind in a place of knowing truth. And if the fear you are feeling is not real, the truth will pierce the lie you are focusing on.

Shift your focus to these basic truths: Are you alive? Yes. Do you exist right now? Yes. At this very moment can you make the decision to eat or drink something? Yes. Can you make the decision to call someone? Yes. Do you have air to breathe? Yes. Do you have a bed or place you can sleep? Yes. Do you know how to laugh? Yes. Are these questions something you can prove? You bet! Can fear eat, drink, breathe, call someone or laugh? No! Therefore it is not real; it is only in your imagination if you allow it to be.

Years ago my then 19-year-old daughter was in Budapest, Hungary, attending a medical class that was only supposed to last six weeks, but the course lasted over three months. She had never lived outside the United States and was used to the freedom of the American way of living. As the three months started to approach, a classmate mentioned she might need to extend her visa, so she decided to go to the American embassy. At the embassy, she was told she had 24 hours to leave the country or the authorities might put her in jail. Fear started to set in. The embassy suggested that my daughter travel to Yugoslavia, and send her passport to an American embassy for a visa to Hungary. When she received it back, she could re-enter the country. You can imagine her fright. All she could think about was that she might be thrown in a Hungarian jail. If you know anything about the jails in Hungary you would not want to be there either. She literally ran back to her little loft where she was staying and called me crying profusely. "I am going to be thrown in jail".

With that opening statement you can imagine how I felt being thousands of miles away in Sacramento, California. There was no way in hell I could fly there in 24-hours to get her out. I had to calm her down before she had a nervous breakdown. When I could get a word in edgewise, I told her everything would be ok. I had to help her collect herself so she could do what was needed to protect herself. So, I started asking her the fundamental questions. I said, "Honey, listen to me and just answer the questions with a yes or no". She said, "Ok, mommy", through her tears. You can imagine how I felt when she called me mommy, oh God!

I began, "Are you in your room now?"
"Yes."
"Are you safe right now at this moment in your room?"
"Yes."
"Do you have food you can eat tonight if you get hungry?"
"Yes."
"We have 24-hours to figure this out, right?"
"Yes."
"Do you have a comfortable bed and pillow to sleep on tonight?"
"Yes." She started to calm down a little.
"Do you have your passport and your credit card with you?"
"Yes."

"Are your suitcases in your room that you can pack right now?"

"Yes."

"So you have the ability to get your belongings together and take a taxi to the airport in the morning and get on a plane back to America, right?"

"Yes."

There was a nine hour time difference, so I said, "While you sleep I will make a reservation for you to get on the first flight back to anywhere in the U.S. You put your phone next to you and I will call you with the flight number, and the time you need to be there."

"Thank you, mommy."

I said to my daughter, "I want you to learn from this. Never allow fear to grip you so that you cannot take action to do what you need to do. Every one of the questions you answered 'yes' to was under your control. You have all of the tools you needed yourself. Always go back to the fundamentals to calm yourself down. Once you are calmed down fill your mind with all the things you love to do, all the people who love you, and know with confidence that you are in control. And as you go through life, put those lovely memories and feelings in a place where you can retrieve them to keep you balanced and focused on your dreams."

Today my daughter is a doctor, and has her own skin care line, which she loves. She still uses this technique when she needs to because she knows her dreams are stronger than anything, and she will not let anything stop her, especially when it is NOT REAL!!!

What is there to Fear? If we are the creators of all that we experience, be it love or fear, then we can also create a life and world filled with love. Fear is a misuse of power. Once we begin to use our power to heal we will see that there is nothing to fear.

Affirmation

What is there to Fear?

- I am fearless before illusion.
- In my right mind I am fearless.
- In my right mind I am in perfect health.
- When I am at peace I am fearless.
- I am fearless when aligned with the remedy.
- I am fearless when I do my homework.
- I am empowered and fearless.
- I am fearlessly honoring myself.
- I am living my best life fearlessly.
- I am giving of myself fearlessly in all my affairs.

CHAPTER EIGHT

Who is in Charge?

Who is in charge of you? It depends on who you are talking to. It could be your husband, your wife, or your mother, father, or guardian. It could also be that you are in charge of yourself. If you are in charge of you then what are you going to do about you? What decisions are you going to make to align yourself with the things that you say you want? When you hear people say, "I want to lose weight", but they are not taking appropriate action to achieve it there is not alignment.

So the questions become: what are you going to do to align yourself with the things you want? What are you willing to do? There are all types of questions you might ask. If you could believe, what could you do? What could you align yourself with? So you just shift the question, change the questions, tweak the question to get to the underlying issue.

Once you determine that you are in charge then what do you want to do? What are you going to think, or say and what action will you take after discovering that you are in charge of you? You realize that I just covered mind, body and soul. It is about walking the walk. Are you walking the walk? I don't feel well, are you walking the walk? Did you change your diet as you said you were going to? Are you getting enough rest? Are you honoring yourself? Are you telling the truth? Are you eating for life?

I have a phrase that I prefer to use, "To thy own self be true." This means to be truthful to yourself. If you are truthful to yourself, you will know the truth, and it's hard to lie to yourself if you know who you are. If it is really true then you should be able to correct it. When you are truthful, you are honoring yourself. When you are honoring a lie, you are trying to prove something. There is nothing to prove. There is no need for a lie when you are so comfortable in your skin it does not matter. We will be truthful to the life we say we want by behaving as such. We will be incongruent with its opposite by behaving as such.

Once we reach a certain age, we realize that we do get to make that choice. No one can tell us what to think for we are in charge of our thoughts. We should be we get to a place where we don't ask anyone to take us as we are because we do not care. The opinions of others become less important. We are content in our own skin. This is the point at which we become more beautiful. We understand that we are more beautiful, confident, and sexy when we are ourselves, comfortable being in our own skin. We become who we are meant to be.

How do you become ok with yourself? So, who is in charge? Is the doctor in charge? Is the government in charge? Is the white man in charge? Is the black man in charge? Is the woman or wife in charge? Who is in charge? The bottom line is, "I am in charge". I am in charge of the way I feel. I get to decide how I am going to feel, not the words you are choosing to use to define me. We say things like, "you make me feel..." but when we say this, we are giving all the responsibility to the other person in the relationship, the husband, the wife, and so on. Who is in charge of your feelings, emotions and happiness? You did not hire your husband to come here to make sure you are having a great day. That is your responsibility. And then you meet in the middle and enjoy each other's company.

The idea is to remind ourselves that we have the power. We have the power to take charge of our thoughts. We should be in charge of our thoughts. Everyone is meant to be in control of their own emotional selves. This is true in all mature relationships. Each individual is responsible for their own feelings and bodies. If we are tuned into the outside world then we are more times than not giving away our power to all the distractions of the world, and blaming the outside world for things not being as we desire. There can be no other way. Because we are too preoccupied, we are listening too much to the outside world. There are too many things that we are picking up on. We must choose to take charge of our emotional state and our thoughts. If we don't, the distractions become our programming, so there is a lack of understanding. I know this works because I have experienced it.

Our insecurity tells people a lot about who we are. For example, the labels on our clothes tell people what we want them to think about us. We want to tell them how much this or that thing cost. It is our insecurity that makes us want to wear designer labels so that someone may think that we are special based on what we are saying because we feel that we are not enough. Our thought then becomes, "Let me put something else out here that might be of interest". So perhaps you tell them what school you went to, what neighborhood you live in, who your parents are, a meaningful conversation that builds relationships.

Celebrities are another example. We know more about these peoples' lives than our own siblings, parents, children, friends etc., even though these are the people we spend most of our lives with. We listen to what they say, we try to dress like them, talk like them, and act like them (no pun intended). This is a clear indication that we are not in charge of our thoughts, feelings and bodies. We then begin to lose our sense of "I am". Isn't it interesting that the majority of us have been conditioned to uphold and uplift celebrities to places of great admiration and god-like status, but for what reason would you want them there? You are idolizing them more so than yourself, and more so than God, who you are calling God for what reason? Yes, all of it is conditioning.

When you pull your energy back from the outside world, you start to take your power back. When you are honoring yourself you are empowering yourself. You are saying: I matter. I am in charge of my feelings. I am not going to allow my feelings to be such that you can say something to hurt my feelings. You cannot hurt my feelings. I can only be hurt if I choose to be hurt. I am in charge of my body. I am in charge of the way I look. For instance, as we age we have a choice: will we age gracefully, and be as fit and healthy as we can be? Or will we ignore the message our bodies give us, and allow poor health to overtake us?

Humans have put everyone in charge except themselves. As you give your power away, you will find it necessary to look outside yourself for healing and your blessing. That is why people look for others to heal them. They look for God to heal them because they have given their power away. The very teachings of religion have disempowered the people, and therein lies the issue. People do not realize that they have the power right now within them to do everything and anything they want, achieve their heart's desire, or whatever they can imagine. They do not know that. And so those who interpret religious teaching have misinterpreted, resulting in the blind leading the blind.

Ask yourself, "Who knows me the best"? The answer will be: I know myself better than anyone else knows me. I know my deepest desires, my deepest thoughts, my deepest secrets. And with that, no one can make better decisions for me than myself. Therefore, if you do not take the initiative to put you in charge of yourself, others will make decisions for you, and those decisions are usually not in your best interest. For this same reason you know what is true and not true about yourself. Aligning yourself with what is true about you and honoring yourself helps you be confident and able to ignore comments that others say or believe about you. You create your own destiny with your decisions. The question is: who do you want to create your destiny? You or others? Who do you want in charge of your life?

Who is in Charge? The moment we are willing to take charge of our lives is the moment that we see that all has been in our control. If our lives are not what we desire then now would be the time to take charge and make a change.

Affirmation

Who is in Charge?

- I have the power to choose the best life has to offer by changing how I feel about it.
- I am the power, the light and the healer.
- I am in charge of what I choose to give my attention to, the thoughts, people and things are all up to me, including what I choose to think about...
  I am choosing love in all my affairs.
- I am the miracle of light and love manifesting out into the world.
- All that I am and all that I need is right here right now.
- I am the miracle worker, healing all I see, touch and think.
- I am in charge of my mind, body and soul.
- I am in charge of my power and how I choose to use it.
  I choose my words wisely, saying words that empower, uplift and inspire me.
- I am a being of light, love and complete awareness.
  Miracles appear before I ask. All is done under grace in divine timing.
- I am in charge of my life and I love it.

CHAPTER NINE

What are you Praying For?

When we think of prayer or praying, it is usually followed by images of hands together, heads bowed down, eyes closed, kneeling beside a bed, an altar, or looking upward towards the heavenly skies while pleading, wishing, for a desired outcome. If only it were so simple. The aforementioned implies that this is indeed the way to pray. I say "so simple" because we have been misled and misguided as to how to pray. What if I were to say that every word is an offering, a seed sown. If we were to think about this for a moment, "reaping what we sow", you realize that every word is a seed. There is no Seed Angel that will tell us what seeds to use, or what seeds will be more prosperous. I say look at your life and what you talk about, as "the apple doesn't fall too far from the tree". I think this phrase helps us understand the importance of our words and prayers. The words we use on a regular basis must bear fruit similar in nature to our experience.

Now that we have a better understanding of prayer, then it is safe to say that everyone is getting what he or she is praying or asking for. People who attend religious services on a regular basis have a life experience similar to that of those who never attend such a service. If we are praying faithfully for a thing and feel as if it is not coming to pass, then we must reexamine the process of praying. In religious text it states, "Therefore I say unto you, all things whatsoever ye pray and ask for, believe that ye have received them, and ye shall have them". If we take this statement and align it with what we talk about on a regular basis, then when we talk about lack of money, time, energy, friends, love, joy, harmony, perfect health and all other lovelessness in our world, I assure you, if these are some of the things you speak of on a regular basis then your life experiences must be similar. For these words are seeds, and you are reaping what you are sowing. What we talk about daily is more times than not what we believe about a person, place or thing. When we adopt this perspective, then it is easy to see that the challenge is to pay attention to what seeds we're sowing with the words we use daily.

If we believe that our words are the prayer, then our lives will soon reflect this new understanding. We then have the power to move mountains. We must believe in what we are praying for and then assume it to be true in our mind, body and soul, or in thought, word and deed. What this means is that there can be no doubt. If we know, then we act like it.

Here's an example: If we are asking for health and continue to smoke, we are not aligned with our desires in mind, body and soul, so how could our prayer be answered? If we desire more money, but complain about not having any, where is the alignment? If we are praying for a partner, yet continue talking about the lack of good men or women out there, it's no wonder we remain single. Because we have practiced the vibration of loneliness, even if a partner does come along they will not stay for our belief in lovelessness is stronger than that of being in love, and it must play itself out. And in no time we will say, "I told you so". I believe that this applies to every aspect of the human experience. Now what are you praying for?

When we pray, we use words or thoughts to convey our desires. Therefore, our everyday words are also delivering up prayer, whether positive or negative. You cannot separate what you want God to hear. If we believe God is omnipotent - able to do anything - then God must be everything and have everything. If this is true, everything already exists in God's world. God knows everything, has everything, IS...everything, right? If this isn't true, then why pray to God (or whatever you believe God to be)? Also, if we believe in God and pray to God, there must be some connection we have with God, such as we must be part of him or why should God hear our prayers?

So, as we pray how do you think God hears us? Where do you think God is? What do you think gives us life? If you say it is the soul or spirit, and if the soul or spirit came from God, then we must have God inside of us. We must be part of the IS... everything. Having God inside us gives us power when we align ourselves with mind, body and soul. And so as we pray, we are not praying to an entity outside us. We are connected to the entity that we are praying to. There can be no separation. Therefore, we should come to an understanding that as we ask for our desires it is done when we are aligned. The timing of the desire to manifest is part of our journey to become aligned. There is a saying, "You have not because you ask not." In your asking you must have certainty that what you ask for is heard. After all, you are the one asking and you are the one connected to your spirit or you would not be alive.

Therefore, in the knowing that your desire has been set forth should you not believe it will manifest? Remember aligning yourself with mind, body and soul is necessary for you to have complete certainty that the desire will start to unfold in the exact best timing. But mind your thoughts because negative thoughts are also sending a strong emotional message or prayer and are easily aligned with you because you know with certainty what you do not like. And certainty is one of the thrusts for manifestation. That is why you hear people say, "Why does this always happen to me?" When you have this complete certainty you will have the confidence to allow God (universe) to present it to you so you do not need to agonize over your prayer. You only need to align yourself and know and know and know that the journey has begun. So I ask you again, "what are you praying for?"

What are you praying for? The thing we are praying for is the thing we see in our experience. The law of the land says, "Ask and you shall receive". Replace the word "ask" with "pray" and you will see what you've been praying for. Every word is a prayer.

Affirmation

What are you Praying for?

- My words, thoughts and actions are aligned with my desires.
- I am one with my desires.
- That which I am seeking is seeking me.
- I am aligning myself with good and goodness defines me.
- I use my words for good.
- My words are the miracle.
- I am the master and the blessing is the healing.
- I am aligned with the end result.
- The best is available to me now.
- My words bring me peace.
- I am willing to open my heart.
- I am willing to surrender to the divine.
- All my prayers are answered promptly.

CHAPTER TEN

One Step at a Time

All we can do is take one step at a time. It doesn't matter what the issue or concern may be. Whether it is good news, or not the news you were hoping for, all is broken down in "one step at a time". If we are given a diagnosis of illness, all we can do is take it one step at a time. The first step is processing the information. How are we going to feel about the information we've just received? How are we going to respond? So, it is important that we understand that all we can do is take one step at a time, even if you hear something dire, like I want a divorce, I'm breaking up with you, I'm having an affair, you're fired, or you have six months to live. It doesn't matter what we hear, because in that moment we have the opportunity to breathe new life into the circumstances, a new perspective. The first step may be to just simply breathe. We have the power to breathe life into any scenario where there is no life. When we find ourselves in such a predicament we must be willing to begin again, to breathe life into the new. We must choose health, love, peace, and power. We must say, "I am open to something more".

First things first. What step are you going to take? Once you decide that then it is moment-to-moment. It is thought-to-thought. It is what you are thinking about at that moment. You are saying, "My first step is to get ahold of my emotions". I am going to tell myself wonderful things, look at goodness, the silver lining, then the right opportunity shall present itself. Your first step could also be changing your thoughts about what you are hearing. Changing your thoughts will change your attitude. Once you change your attitude and you are holding that vibration long enough, your body must follow. And that goes back to who's in charge. Your thoughts first and then your feelings will follow. You will forever take one step at a time. That is all you can take, so you are not going to look at the experience as a whole. It is only going to be one day at a time, holding your vibration in the goodness, being in alignment with the end result in mind, body and soul. Being in line with the mind, body and soul. It is the process. Everyone has this present moment in time. Yesterday is gone and tomorrow doesn't exist yet. Now is what counts.

Just think about the few moments before you heard some unpleasant news and your world was turned upside down. Everything was status quo – the same. Then in an instant you changed everything in your core or alignment of mind, body, and soul with negative emotions from reacting to the unpleasant news. It is the emotions that cause a mind-shifting phenomena which freezes the ability to think clearly, to act clearly, be able to heal yourself, and robs you of your energy! This amplifies the emotions being expressed, which is what we do not want. Therefore, the first step is to shift your emotions to think upon something pleasant. It does not matter what you have to think about. Just something that makes you laugh or feel good. I mean anything, and hold that thought that makes you feel better. Get a funny movie, listen to your favorite music. If this doesn't work, rest your mind by taking a nap, but you must shift your emotions.

Putting positive input in your mind will allow you to clear your mind of negative emotions. When you clear your mind other steps will unfold for what you should do. It is still one step at a time, but we must put our mind in a state that can capture what the next step will be, and the next and the next. Every time you start to go emotionally negative repeat whatever process you did before that made you feel better. Emotions are one of the strongest gifts we have. Whether negative or positive, it is powerful what they can do to your mind, body and soul. It is, in essence, a barometer to let you know if you are in a good place or not. The stronger positive emotions you have, the stronger the ability your mind will have to capture inspiration from your spirit, and be in alignment for miracles to happen.

As the steps unfold, the process of what you need to do and why this happened will unfold. You will also be shown a new path that is better for you that could not have unfolded unless you learned the power of who you are and what you are made up of. Most people who have gone through very unpleasant circumstances and have changed their outlook with positive emotions say they would not have changed the experience because of who they have become. Now I know it is hard to see the end when you are in it, but what if you told yourself that the whole mess was going to reveal something special to you? Would you view the experience a little differently at the beginning?

One Step at a Time: There is a process to any and everything we do, we must be willing to take the first step in the right direction. The first step will always be the first step. You can't go wrong by taking it.

Affirmation Ten

One Step at a Time

- I am present in every moment.

- I am willing to do more, to be more every day in every way.

- I am the change that I desire by being it now.

- I am willing to see the good and to walk toward it.

- I walk with joy to a happy ending, right here, right now.

- I appreciate and anticipate the best.

- I am putting my best foot forward with every step.

- I am healed with every step; I walk with conviction.

- I shall take my first step with confidence.

- I walk in grace on the path of healing...for all starts with one step.

CHAPTER ELEVEN

Dropping the Past: What is the Past?

We experience life in the present moment. It is all we have and anything else is the past, for the future is a thought/breath away. When we speak of our past it is usually referring to anytime other than the present experience, be it yesterday or twenty years ago. It will be what we want it to be. We can choose to learn from our past or use it as a crutch that ties us to some emotional trauma that we haven't been willing to process. It doesn't matter what we feel we've experienced. I am sure if we look hard enough we will find those that have lived through the very thing, in that moment, we believed was unbearable. I say it's very important to give careful consideration and contemplation to our past and the energy we give to it on a daily basis. This is accomplished by paying close attention to what we talk about. Is it an unhealed experience, something we haven't been willing to let go of? The past has no power but that which we assign to it. In every moment there is an opportunity to drop the past if we are willing to. When we have some emotional connection to our past we will talk about it giving it power/energy, calling it forth into our present and future experiences. It becomes a self-fulfilling prophecy. It doesn't matter if the thing we are reminiscing about is from a place of love or fear, we are destined to repeat it. This concept alone should inspire us to learn to process our emotions and move forward. The past is just our thoughts about one thing or another.

REPEATING PATTERNS FROM YOUR PAST

The past is dead. There is no life in it but that which we breathe into it by talking about it, complaining about it. If we share from a place of empowerment, and are inspired by our story and those who hear it are reminded of something more, then I say the past is worth repeating (sharing).

One example might be someone dealing with addiction. In some circles we will always be hearing about the recovering addict. I believe it's a fine line to walk for when does the recovering becomes the recovered? Isn't that the purpose? That we might be a healed and empowered spiritual being, to be more than what we once believed possible for ourselves? If we are breathing life into all that we are saying, are we not bringing forth the very condition that we are trying to move away from? Would it not be better to say, "I am loving myself in a way that supports a healthy lifestyle, fueling me with inspiration and loving energy on a daily basis?"

THE PAST DOES NOT DEFINE WHO YOU ARE OR YOUR FUTURE

The past does not define who we are, or what we will be or are capable of being. Holding onto the past affects every area of our lives. How much power are we going to give to the past? We must begin to use our past as a springboard into our future. The possibilities for our future are limitless. Whatever we believe becomes possible. We must be willing to dream, to use our imagination to manifest the best life has to offer. It is when we let go of the past that we are free to create a new present and a better future.

We are special and unique beings filled with limitless possibilities with the power to change our world. I say we should rise above our past and give ourselves the opportunity to be successful in all that we do, for all flows through us and to us. It is up to each person to reevaluate their past and release it.

Dropping the Past: If we desire something more, something better than what was, then we must be willing to let go of what used to be, and imagine what and how it should be and can be. This is possible when we become free from our past.

Affirmation Eleven

Dropping the Past

- I am honoring myself in every moment of my life.
- I am honoring myself today for today is a new beginning.
- I am honoring the person I am and meant to be.
- I am honoring myself for making new choices.
- I am honoring myself for telling a new story.
- The past is powerless in the awareness of the present.
- I shall use the past as a springboard to live my best life.
- I shall use the past as a teaching tool to help heal myself.
- The past is over, the present is here and the future is the best I can imagine.
- I am looking for the love in my past experiences for it has shaped me into the person I am today.

CHAPTER TWELVE

Forgiveness

Forgiveness is defined as a conscious, deliberate decision to release feelings of resentment or vengeance toward a person. Forgiveness does not always involve such strong emotions like resentment or vengeance. I think it also applies to any level of disharmony, an unhealed emotion that we may want to release, an emotion triggered by a past experience that is less inspiring, bringing up feelings of sadness and disempowerment. I believe that it must start with us - the individual. We must be willing to forgive ourselves first.

We are starting to realize the impact that our unhealed emotions have on our physical body. Some believe that physical ailments may stem from our unhealed emotional selves. This is in alignment with the need to forgive. We must also consider that it doesn't matter if the unforgiven person wants to be forgiven. The one holding the unhealed emotions shall be the reciprocator of those feelings. The would-be perpetrator more times than not couldn't care less about our feelings. We have all we need within us to experience the closure necessary to move on with our lives, for the person may never give us the answer that will justify their words or actions. The same process applies to them as well, for they must be willing to forgive themselves or they will suffer the same fate. Our body is affected by our emotional energy, be it negative or positive. The other person's body is not affected by our anger and resentment, or our unwillingness to forgive. We can now see why it is important that we let go and release the unhealed. If we do not choose to release this emotional poison, then we will find some residual effects playing themselves out in our lives or our bodies, and in some cases both.

I stated that the first person we must forgive is ourselves for any and everything that we did or did not do. We have the power to shift our perception of our emotional trauma and drama from one of powerlessness to one of complete power and emotional freedom. The emotional energy of not forgiving can ruin our lives if we allow it. When we begin to look at our emotions as energy then we know the importance of releasing this negative energy. It is important to forgive in order to process and release negative energy.

By now you know that we are beings of energy and spirit (energetic/spiritual beings), and that the spirit is energy, which makes us energy as well. As energetic/spiritual beings, any deviation from positive to negative energy, such as when we have negative emotions, disrupts our balance. This concept means we do not want to store unhealed energy in our body or in our energetic field. Because anything stored in our energetic field will soon become our physical ailment. If we hold on to anger, resentment, hatred, fear, jealousy, all that emotional poison will eventually take a toll on our physical being. Forgiveness is about loving yourself more than the situation because we do not want the pain to continue to hurt us. That's like asking someone to do it again. Let it go because you want it as far from you as possible. Cut those chains and get out of jail! Free....yourself. Do not let the past be your present.

Forgiveness is a choice we must be willing to make. The person who has wronged us does not need to make that choice because we have to carry that energy until we are wise enough to process and release it. Forgiveness doesn't mean that we must have dinner with that person. We forgive for ourselves. We are the benefactor of this new positive energy flowing through our body. Aspire to a new level of being and say, "I no longer want to be tied to this energetic imbalance. I want to feel light and free." We cannot fly or soar in this world while holding on to resentment and unhealed emotions. We cannot be the best we can be by holding onto resentment. We cannot thrive in our personal relationships, or any other for that matter, when we are angry and upset about something or someone we haven't forgiven.

When we do not forgive, the person or situation that is bothering us remains unaffected. They do not care. We are hoping that they feel bad for their part in our unhappiness, that they might experience some type of remorse. We hope that they care enough about us to say that they are sorry. But what if they don't? More importantly, when we are holding on to unhealed emotions the thing we are thinking about, the unhealed thing we're worried about, becomes repeated in our present experiences. We say, "I can't believe this person behaved this way and did such-and-such." In this emotional energetic alignment we are calling on that experience to meet someone similar, and repeat the very thing we are trying to avoid. We will get what we focus on, and the cycle repeats itself once again, because we are sowing the seed of the unhealed scenario. We are sowing the seed of anger, bitterness or the role of a victim. The very fact that we are holding on to it means that we are tuned into it. We may think that if we forgive, we condone the person. The fact is that when we do not forgive, and hold on to being angry at the person or situation, we are destined to repeat it. So, not only is it important to forgive for our mental, emotional and spiritual wellbeing, but we also have an opportunity to break a pattern or cycle that keeps us tied to a life level that no longer serves us.

The moment will come when we know why we continue to attract this type of situation, this type of man, this type of neighbor, this type of boss. And in our religious teaching it says, "love thy neighbor as thyself", but most of us do not love ourselves and are not willing to forgive ourselves, so how can we forgive another? How can we offer forgiveness to another when we haven't offered it to ourselves? We can only see where we are. If we are judgmental of ourselves, we will attract someone who needs to judge. It is important to let go. It is about forgiving, having the willingness to practice and believe that we no longer want to be tied to this emotional baggage.

We must be willing to disengage from all that no longer empowers us. Although years may have passed, the energy is ageless and timeless, and feels like yesterday. It will dictate our behavior, even as we are saying someone has done us wrong or has mistreated or disrespected us. This person may have moved on with their life, while we remain stuck until we are ready to forgive. It is similar to a mother saying to a child, "You are horrible. You are never going to amount to anything". The child grows up and is no longer in the presence of the mother, but they still behave as if their mother is there. Not only do they behave like the mother is there, they are going to attract people that are like their mother. They will attract a partner who will tell them they are worthless, and so on, and all areas of your life will be a reflection of the unforgiveness. May we be willing to see the importance of forgiving "self" first.

Forgiveness: We must be willing to forgive ourselves first before we can forgive anyone else. It is true when you hear someone say forgiveness is the gift we give ourselves.

Affirmations Twelve

Forgiveness

- I forgive myself for not knowing.
- I forgive myself for not listening to myself.
- I forgive myself not honoring myself.
- I forgive myself for not letting go.
- I forgive myself for not being honest.
- I forgive myself for not trusting myself.
- I forgive myself for not living my best life.
- I forgive myself for not making better choices.
- I forgive myself for not saying no.
- I forgive myself for playing small.

CHAPTER THIRTEEN

Redefine Yourself

I t is important to redefine ourselves - a check point. We must be willing to take a close look at our lives and see who we have become, and decide if it is who we really are. Are we the person we want to be, or are we a product of what others want us to be? How are we being to ourselves and those around us? Are we bringing something positive to our lives and the lives of those around us? Are we the person we say we want to be? Are we living the life we say we want to live?

In every moment we have an opportunity to begin again. A woman discovered she had cancer and knew she needed to make immediate changes in her world if she was going to heal herself from this disease. She said, "I need to change my thoughts". In that moment she began to redefine herself as a person who is now cancer free. Everything needed to change from her thoughts, to her eating habits, and of course, her attitude towards cancer. We must be willing to say, "I am going to decide who I want to be in this world. I desire to be a person of peace, strength and compassion. I am a person with perfect health, an energetic person. I am a vibrant spiritual being living a life aligned with the best life I can imagine - in mind, body and soul". It is in this moment that we began to redefine ourselves, our lives.

Once we decide that we want something more from life and in life, we must then ask, "Who do I need to be to get this thing? What thoughts do I need to think in order to become this type of person"? Then we must move to action to become the person we desire to be. We cannot redefine ourselves by doing the things we've done before. The definition of insanity is doing the same thing over and over again and expecting different results. We will not and cannot change our lives thinking the same thoughts that created the situation, illness, lackluster environment we call our work, home, relationship and state of health. If we find ourselves in a state of declining health we must be willing to do the best we can to first change what we are thinking in regard to our health. Our attitude towards an issue makes all the difference.

As we move through life without question we find that life is ok, and that there is not much we can do for ourselves; we do not ask much of ourselves or of life. We have taken a stance that it is what it is. If this is the case we will not question our state of health and our life level, for we feel powerless to make a change. The good news is if you are reading these words, this book, then it's safe to say that you believe that you have the power to redefine yourself and your life.

Redefining yourself changes your way of thinking. Your mind is a new and so is your outlook in the way you look at the world, the way you look at your health, and the way you see yourself. It is about a change in consciousness. That is the redefining moment. The beautiful thing is you get to decide who you want to be. You get to decide. You get to decide if you are going to be a cranky person who dreads getting up in the morning, or if you are going to be a happy person who is excited about life no matter what it looks like. You have the power to redefine every aspect of it.

Change your consciousness. That is the purpose of redefining our thought process. When you redefine your life you become aligned with the thing you desire. That is the determining moment. It is what you are going to say, how you are going to respond, that will determine the outcome. In that moment you get to redefine who you are, who you have been, what you believe about yourself. You get to decide. You can say in that moment, "I no longer believe it", and then you have a clean slate. And you get to decide what you want to believe. And that's the beauty and the power. And that's the truth. Redefining yourself is necessary for this process.

When you come to a place of re-examining your life, there is usually some catalyst that made you ask if this is what you want, where you want to be.

Whatever it may be, it motivated you to re-examine your life. After going through a divorce, I realized that my inner being had truly been suffocated and controlled. Every day I wrestled with my spirit, knowing that my situation was not right. Being of strong mind and will, I squashed those feelings by living a fast-paced life, taking care of business instead of taking the time to reflect and deal with my personal life. And when it got to a point that I had to examine myself, I knew I was not happy. I figured I could wait until the time was right to make a decision about what to do. But when I started to examine my life, I created momentum. As I thought about rectifying my situation, the excitement of doing the right thing, of being the person I truly am, took over as if I had jet engines on my back. The positive flow of energy that went through my mind as I finally understood my true desire to move in the direction I wanted to move in, was unstoppable. I had activated something. It was my positive emotions and the universe heard it. My conscious decision to change came from my soul not allowing me to continue in this situation. We are more than our minds, and our spirit knows our signature or the vibrations that are best for us. When we are true to ourselves, we will follow what makes us happy, which will put our body, mind, and soul in alignment. Once in alignment, you can do anything because the universe/God will guide you by bringing what you need at the right time to make all the decisions you need and live life to its fullest. I was going to overcome my negative situation, and never allow myself to squash my emotions again. From that moment on, I have been redefining my life in ways I could not have possibly understood before. It has been the most exhilarating, fantastic feeling to allow myself the joy of feeding my spirit with joyous feelings, and seeing what's next for me.

Redefining Yourself: Every moment is an opportunity to redefine ourselves, to begin again. We get another chance for something more. If we are unhappy with something then we must redefine what it means, and keep moving forward.

Affirmation Thirteen
Redefining Yourself

- In every moment, with every breath I am redefining myself.
- I am redefining my mind, body and soul.
- I am redefining my health and wellbeing.
- I am redefining to be one with balance.
- I am redefining to be one with peace.
- I am redefining to be one with grace.
- I am redefining myself as peace, love and light.
- I am redefining myself as the self-healer.
- I am redefining myself as the power, the oneness.
- I am redefining myself as pure love.
- I am redefining that I am the all-knowingness and connectedness.
- I am redefining my thoughts about my body, life, and world.
- I am redefining my emotional state, my emotional self, and releasing all that there is to the great divine (or collective consciousness).

CHAPTER FOURTEEN

Free Your Mind

When it comes to freeing your mind, there are two things to consider. You can free your mind when there is complete silence and stillness for meditation or prayer. There is another freeing of mind when we let go of a belief that prevents growth or precludes other ideas. When we believe that we know something how can we expect anything other than what we know to be true. So this has to be our belief system. Freeing our mind is saying: I am no longer going to hold onto something that is out of my control or field of expertise, for I do not know what is going to happen. I shall remain open to the goodness and the endless possibilities and opportunities that may be the very thing I need. I am open for healing, to finding a place of peace from within so that I may be guided to the solution. I do not want to clutter my mind. I do not wish to preoccupy my mind or my thoughts with things that do not serve me. I do not want to use my mind to talk about the weather because I have no control over it. I do not want to tune into the masses with their self-talk and beliefs for it becomes my life experiences, my beliefs. If you hear something long enough you will start to believe it.

Some people base their attitude on the weather. If it's sunny out then it's a beautiful day. We hear the news announcer's opinion about the day based on the amount of clouds in the sky. They may describe the day as gloomy. If we listen to such talk we begin to believe cloudy days are gloomy days. Our minds become cluttered with useless information that we have come to believe as truth, and will repeat at the perfect opportunity to get others to see it as they do.

Free your mind of any heaviness and adopt a childlike attitude of knowing that the day will be the day. It is up to you what you do with it. I wish to free my mind that I may dream a new dream, tell a new story, and use my power for good that I might heal myself first and then be an example for those around me. I might be the shining light in the darkness that someone else might find their way to healing, to a better life. I shall free myself from my past, for in my present I can design the ideal experience by freeing my mind.

Someone once said that thinking slows down intelligence. Think about that. Thinking slows down intelligence because intelligence is a movement of being and flows through all things, including us. Thinking is figuring out and doing instead of knowing. That is the difference. We should be in a place of being, where we know where to be, how to be, and who to be. And that is the purpose of freeing the mind. We must be the things that we want to be - be nice, be healthy, be peaceful, be it. So it is the feeling - just be, not just do. I am going to take over that Nike slogan: instead of "just do it", "just be". Be whatever you feel you are comfortable being. That is the thing: BE IT!!

It is necessary to free your mind because that is where the answers are. When we free our minds of the day's concerns and find ourselves preoccupied with the dishes, playing with the dog, planting flowers, dancing, or doing yoga, our minds are clutter-free, and in this space the answers come. It slips right in there when we are preoccupied with something else, when the mind is quiet.

When answers come the ego will rationalize the acceptance of the answer. The ego speaks loudest and has a tendency to defend its position, whether right or wrong. Within a free mind there is none of that, because there is a level of awareness and knowingness that doesn't need to defend the truth, if we are aware of truth. Only those who are not aware of truth will try to defend it. Truth does not need us to defend it. It is there and stands on its own.

The purpose is to free our minds of all the useless chatter. With a free mind we will experience small miracles happening on a daily basis all day long.

We will find ourselves in the right place at the right time. We get in the right line at the right time. We will go to the person at the counter who is going to give us the best service ever, who is going to give us exactly what we are looking for, in spite of what we may have heard. With a clear mind we know what action to take. We have a worry-free attitude for we know that we are now communing with a place of peace from within. Our thoughts then become in alignment with grace and goodness.

So it is about understanding how to use your power, and you will use your power when you have a free mind. You can use your power when your mind is free because your mind is not competing with the spirit where all knowledge and power comes from. So you have to understand that you have power first of all. You are the power. You are it. Do you realize that the universe does not move until you are offering something? It does not move until you are offering a feeling or a thought, and it is up to you what you are feeling or thinking. If you are tuned into the outside world you will have a cluttered mind. Your mind cannot be free if you are listening to the world. When you have a free mind and are aligned with the goodness, then all answers are available. You will be aligned as one with all, not resisting the gift of who you are, you will just be it.

Free Your Mind: We will discover the answers in the silence of our mind, where the mind is not preoccupied with worry and problem-solving. Lighten up and listen, and in the emptiness of your mind the answers await.

Affirmation

Free your Mind

- My mind is in tune with the divine.
- I am free to imagine the best the world has to offer.
- There is clarity in a free mind.
- My thoughts are clear and precise. I get what I focus on.
- In every moment there is freedom to change.
- In every moment I am free to begin again.
- My mind has no boundaries.
- My mind is clutter-free.
- I reside in a space of emotional freedom.
- My thoughts are free to heal my body.

CHAPTER FIFTEEN

Quiet Time

What is quiet time, and why is it necessary to make time for it? The definition will mean something different to everyone. I wanted to share this idea because we must be willing to find time to rejuvenate to recharge our spiritual battery.

Quiet time doesn't necessarily mean that we need to sit in front of an altar in the lotus position. We must first realize that it is necessary to make time for silence. This is more about the inner chatter that keeps our mind busy - too busy to experience peace and quiet. This state can be accomplished while doing anything you love. We must be willing to incorporate this practice into our daily routine, especially if we find that our daily routine pulls us away from this space. I'm sure some will say, "Who has time for that"? To this I say, if we feel we are too busy to make time to rejuvenate our spiritual energy then all shall suffer - work, health, family and friends - for over time we become exhausted emotionally, spiritually and physically, and who has time for that? We will not know the importance of this if we are plugged into the TV and the pettiness of the world. We will give more credence to a world that is filled with doom and gloom, and this then becomes our preoccupation. We then hear some say, I can't stick my head in the sand and pretend that nothing is happening, or I can't see the world through rose-colored glasses. They talk as though their pity and awareness makes a difference to the resolution. Unbeknownst to them is that the plight of mankind is perpetuated by their need to point it out from a place of fear and hopelessness, creating more of the same.

I know we want to help the world become a more peaceful place. We will believe this to be the case when we tune into the horrors of the world. If we are tuned into love in our own world, personal experience, then we begin to see the world through new eyes - those of love and peace - because we have a better understanding of ourselves and know the power we possess, and from this place all is well in the world. We then remember the power and importance of quiet time. Marianne Williamson noted that you can't solve the problem at the level of the problem. I alluded to this in the previous paragraph. If we are complaining about something, we do not help to solve it for the mindset that created it will not be the same mind that finds the solution. It is within the quiet mind that we find the answers. I am not talking about meditation and what most equate to quiet time. I am suggesting that we take our thoughts off the issue and put them on something that we would prefer to be thinking about, perhaps something that we may get lost in while doing it - drawing, painting, bike riding, gardening, reading a nice book - anything that will bring a level of peace and quiet from within.

Everyone has experienced those moments when we were lost in the zone - where the task becomes automatic and effortless, and we can do this without thinking. Getting into this space is so simple that you can do it while doing the mundane, such as taking a shower, mowing the lawn, taking a nap. Haven't you lost yourself while doing the dishes and reminiscing about dinner and a conversation you had? You forget what you're doing. You lose yourself in that moment and before long the entire kitchen is clean because you were not standing there complaining. At that moment, you were aligned with being, allowing yourself to just do what you were doing. You were so in the moment that the spirit radiated peace and quiet within, which is the true you. Isn't that beautiful? In Being (quiet time), there is peace because you are not bothered that no one is helping you clean the kitchen.

Some people may be afraid to experience quiet time, or to intentionally set out to do something to achieve this state. We hear religious teachings say, "The answer comes over a calm sea and the calm sea is a quiet mind." In the moment of complete surrender we find what we are looking for. The answers are in the quiet space. We can't find our keys and look up and down and all around for them, and still we can't find them. Then, in the moment of surrender, we get an idea where we might find them, and often it is a place we thoroughly checked moments before. What is the thing you love doing that pulls you away from this world into the quiet spaces of your mind? We owe it to ourselves to make time to be quiet.

Quiet Time: We discover all we need to know when we are willing to just be quiet. Quiet time takes practice. Sometimes we need to be quiet and listen to others, but first we must listen to ourselves, and make time for quiet time

Affirmation

Quiet Time

- I am more energized after a few moments of peace and quiet.
- I am looking for opportunities to experience more peace of mind.
- I am more powerful with a clear and peaceful mind.
- I find more clarity in my quiet time.
- I make the opportunity for quiet time.
- All my answers are available in the quiet spaces of my mind.
- I am now making time on a daily basis to be quiet.
- There is peace to be had in the midst of chaos.
- I have the power to quiet my mind at will.
- There is balance in silence for all is well.

CHAPTER SIXTEEN

Living in Grace

Grace is alignment. It is alignment in truth. Grace is being aware that we are connected to all there is - God/the source energy - that of love and light, being our authentic selves. In these moments, we no longer see ourselves as separate from everything and everyone around us. We begin to offer better feelings and thoughts towards ourselves and those around us. As we offer better feelings our positive emotions make us feel more restored, fueling more positive and joyous thoughts, and the cycle continues as the universe cannot resist aligning with our innermost desires, without us saying a word. And so we see that the universe is giving us the best we can imagine in every given moment, and we start to see the role we play in the world.

Grace is being in alignment with synchronistic events. This is how you know you are in alignment. As more synchronistic events appear, your innermost being or higher self is being demonstrated. Grace leads and takes control of our lives and the power we possess by setting up the perfect scenarios that will take us on a journey of bliss and ease. It is where things unfold as we wish because we know how to express our power through positive emotions, to live the life we say we want to live - creating our synchronistic events based on what we are thinking about. The more we express joy, love and excitement, the greater the strength of our power will be to be aligned with grace.

There is nothing that is happening outside of us that we aren't a part of. We have something to do with everything. EVERYTHING!!! Perfect timing is our thoughts. Our thoughts align ourselves with what we call perfect timing. When thought and energy align, we are allowed the privilege to experiencing what are called synchronistic events - our thoughts and feelings do just that.

We hear, "Oh God did this, God set this up. See how God has treated my husband because he has been mean to me". Do you really think that was God's doing? When I hear this, I know that this is a person that is not willing to take responsibility for his or her life. We don't need to create a God outside of ourselves. What we have to do is look at our experiences and we will see that we truly are reaping what we sow. That's how they ended up being aligned in marriage, and then hating each other for being the very thing they are. This happens when you do not honor yourself first, which gives tacit permission for your partner to mistreat you. There is no grace in this.

When we look out into the world, we find it is beautifully orchestrated so that we might have the opportunity to see who we've become by our life experiences. We discover this through the type of partner we are married to - actually all of our relationships fall under this category. It is an opportunity to see where we may need to fine tune our evolutionary process and progress - to see if we are being the person we say we want to be.

When we are in Grace we remember who we are. We are at ease, at peace. We do not worry because all we need to do is put our attention on goodness and the goodness comes. If we are capable of holding our attention on something long enough, it will come. This is happening if we are aware of it or not, so why not use our power for good? Synchronistic events are the natural occurrence for each and every one of us being tuned in, it cannot not happen because it's the nature of our being and the universe.

When we are aligned, it does not matter where we are. Because the person that is living in Beverly Hills is still using the same power as the person living in the slums of Los Angeles. Both are using their power in two different ways – both are in grace – both have access to the same power. If you are looking to your partner to provide grace, that is not grace. There is nothing graceful about it. Grace is about being who you want to be - being your authentic self.

Grace is simply the full circle of everything we have talked about in this book. Grace reveals itself to us when we are aligned in mind, body and soul, and allowing ourselves the understanding of who we are. The power of grace is shown through synchronistic events being so gracious in revealing our desires, whether we have asked or not, in such perfect timing that many may call it a miracle. The soft touch of grace is the most powerful gift of all that the universe presents to all of us. Everything from moving mountains, to parting the sea, to finding a parking space up front in a packed parking lot, to finding a new job, healings, a partner, and as small as helping us find our keys when we have misplaced them. It makes sense when you think how we manifest desires. When we align ourselves by understanding that we are ultimately responsible for our thoughts and have the ability to change our thoughts, and allow our emotions to be those of joy, passion, and excitement, and know that fear is only an illusion, then we know alignment will follow. The more we become aligned, the more we stay aligned. The frequency sent out is more of a match with the true nature of who we are, our true inner core. The reason for this is that those positive uplifting emotions give off a vibration that is the frequency of your core natural self, which aligns you to your desires.

Therefore, we are ultimately in charge of deciding what we want to think, who we want to be and that it is US who makes those decisions. We must choose wisely what we focus on because that focus becomes our prayers and thoughts that are offered up to the universe for manifestation. Therefore, we need to focus our thoughts on the now, for there is only NOW. Whether you chose to believe that the past is gone, the future has not arrived, or all time happens simultaneously, now is what gets processed in the universe. Everything is in the now and so you can only do one step at a time, not looking back. Forgive yourself to free your mind, and allow yourself quiet time for inspirational thoughts from your higher self to flow to you. Embody that you are one with all, you are the "I am", you are the conduit for the full connection of manifestation when you are aligned mind, body and soul. You will see how grace manifests your desires through synchronicity over and over again.

And so my friends as I wrote this book, I too was learning, reexamining my thoughts and understanding that certain events – good and bad – in my life, were of my doing, that I attracted these events. The change in my life came about by writing health books for a new company I started called Optimal Life. In every book and section I always repeated in the middle and at the end, "Live life to the fullest the way life was meant to be lived because you deserve an optimal life!!!" Well, when you repeat that for about five years in a row it starts to affect you, and you start to ask yourself the question, "Am I living life the way I want it – to the fullest? Is this it? What is inside of me that causing me to ask these questions? And when I answered the question from my true inner core – my soul – I started to move in the direction of who I am, which brought me to where I am now. WOW, what a lesson learned. Sometimes I think it would have been nice if someone had given me this formula in my childhood, but it was the experience of the journey up to this point that allowed me to understand. Therefore, I realize the timing of the unfolding of who I am was in perfect timing.

And as I close, I have a question to ask you: Are you listening to your inner voice, your soul and spirit to know...what's inside?

Living in Grace: We move through life pushing through to the next thing, trying to make this thing or that thing happen. Grace is remembering that we need not do anything; we only need to BE and all will flow to us.

Affirmation

Living in Grace

- I am living in grace.
- All my affairs unfold in grace.
- I am grateful in every moment with all I encounter.
- I am in grace with clear intentions to do so.
- Grace is the way to happiness.
- Grace gives me forgiveness and love.
- When I am in grace, I am always in the right place at the right time.
- Living in grace brings forth blessings.
- I am the balance, beauty and the grace.
- I am grateful for all I need.
- I am grateful in the world and the world responds accordingly.
- I resolve my issues with grace.
- The solution is found in grace.

Other Titles by Christine Lee-Schaffer

Optimal Life: The Essentials of Diabetes (2010)
Available as a book, or book and two-disc
DVD set. Also available in Spanish.

Optimal Life: The Essentials of Breast Cancer (2011)
Book and DVD, in collaboration with Dr. Ernie Bodai.

Optimal Life: The Essentials of Asthma (2012)
Available as a book, or book and two-disc
DVD set. Also available in Spanish.

Optimal Life: The Essentials of Insulin (2013)

Optimal Life: The Essentials of Hypertension (2013)

Optimal Life: The Essentials of Cold and Flu (2014)
Available as a DVD.

Optimal Life: How to Use Weight Machines at the Gym (2014)
DVD in collaboration with Travis Grosjean.

Optimal Life: The Essentials of High Cholesterol (2015)

Available at
www.optimalife.net
iBookstore
Amazon Kindle
Barnes & Noble
Kobo
Baker & Taylor

Contact the author at
info@optimalife.net